KIDNEY DISEASE DIET FOODS CHART FOR SENIORS ON STAGE 3

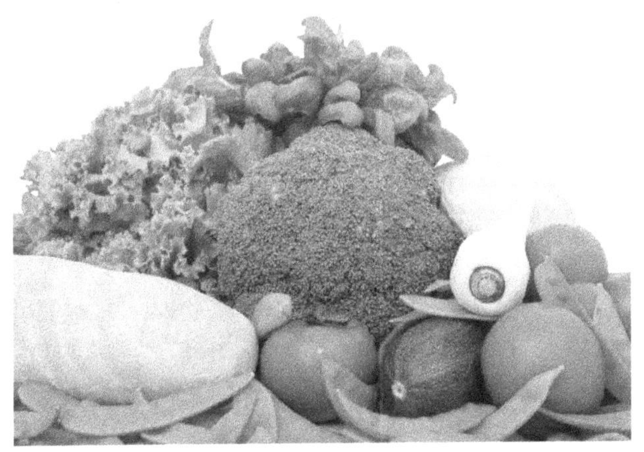

The Complete Guide to Stage 3 Kidney Disease Diet: Unleashing a Collection of Recipes and Food Lists with Low Sodium, Potassium, and Phosphorus

Felicia O. Pace

For more evidence-based and approved nutrition books similar to this, explore my Amazon store. HERE

Table of Contents

INTRODUCTION

As individuals age, the importance of maintaining optimal health becomes increasingly significant, particularly for those managing chronic conditions such as Stage 3 Chronic Kidney Disease (CKD). Seniors in Stage 3 CKD require a specialized and well-balanced diet to support kidney function, manage symptoms, and enhance overall well-being. The kidney disease diet for seniors at this stage focuses on regulating key nutrients like sodium, potassium, phosphorus, and protein while ensuring adequate fluid intake. This carefully crafted dietary approach aims to slow the progression of kidney dysfunction, alleviate associated complications, and enhance the quality of life for older individuals.

Understanding Stage 3 CKD:
In Stage 3 CKD, the kidneys exhibit moderate impairment in their ability to filter waste and excess fluids from the blood. While kidney function is compromised, individuals may not always experience noticeable symptoms. However, it is crucial to implement dietary modifications to alleviate stress on the kidneys and maintain health.

The Significance of Diet in Stage 3 CKD:
Diet plays a pivotal role in managing Stage 3 CKD. A kidney-friendly diet for seniors in this stage is designed to mitigate further damage to the kidneys, regulate electrolyte balance, and control blood pressure. Additionally, it helps manage associated conditions such as diabetes, which can contribute to kidney complications. By adopting a kidney disease diet, seniors can positively impact their overall health, reduce the risk of complications, and maintain a better quality of life.

For individuals in Stage 3 of kidney disease, it's important to limit or avoid certain foods that may contribute to the progression of kidney dysfunction. Here's a list of foods to limit or avoid in a kidney disease diet:

1. High-Sodium Foods:
    1. Processed foods (canned soups, frozen meals, processed meats)
    2. Restaurant/fast-food meals
    3. Pickled and canned vegetables
    4. Salted snacks (chips, pretzels)

2. High-Potassium Foods:
    1. Bananas
    2. Oranges and orange juice
    3. Potatoes (especially baked and sweet potatoes)
    4. Tomatoes and tomato-based products
    5. Spinach and other high-potassium greens

3. High-Phosphorus Foods:
    1. Dairy products (milk, cheese, yogurt)
    2. Nuts and seeds
    3. Colas and other dark sodas

4. Processed meats (bacon, sausage, hot dogs)
5. Chocolate and cocoa products

4. High-Protein Foods:
   1. Red meat (beef, lamb, pork)
   2. Processed meats (sausages, hot dogs, bacon)
   3. Organ meats (liver, kidney)
   4. High-protein supplements

5. High-Phosphorus Additives:
   1. Phosphoric acid-containing beverages (colas)
   2. Packaged foods with phosphate additives (read labels)
   3. Baking powder and baking soda

6. High-Potassium Salt Substitutes:
   1. Salt substitutes containing potassium chloride

7. Excessive Fluid Intake:
   - Monitoring fluid intake is crucial, but excessive restriction can lead to dehydration.

8. Certain Fruits:
   - Limit intake of high-potassium fruits like bananas, oranges, and melons.

9. Certain Vegetables:
- Limit high-potassium vegetables like potatoes, tomatoes, and spinach.

10. Whole Grains:
- Whole grains can contain higher levels of phosphorus; moderation is advised.

11. High-Sugar Foods:
- Excessive intake of sugary foods and beverages.

12. Alcohol:
- Excessive alcohol consumption can impact kidney function.

It's essential for individuals in Stage 3 kidney disease to work closely with healthcare professionals, particularly a registered dietitian or nutritionist, to develop a personalized dietary plan. The goal is to manage nutrients, especially sodium, potassium, phosphorus, and protein, while maintaining overall health. Regular monitoring and adjustments to the diet may be necessary based on individual health status and laboratory results. Always consult with healthcare professionals for personalized advice tailored to specific health needs

Comprehensive Dietary guidelines for stage 3 kidney disease

Dietary guidelines for individuals with Stage 3 kidney disease focus on managing key nutrients, especially sodium, potassium, phosphorus, and protein, to support kidney function and overall health. It's important to note that individual dietary needs can vary, and these guidelines should be adapted based on specific health conditions and recommendations from healthcare professionals, including dietitians or nephrologists. Here's a comprehensive set of dietary guidelines for Stage 3 kidney disease:

1. Sodium Management:
    2. Aim for a low-sodium diet to help control blood pressure and fluid balance.
    3. Limit processed and packaged foods, which often contain high levels of sodium.
    4. Use herbs, spices, and lemon juice for flavor instead of salt.
    5. Choose fresh, whole foods and cook at home to have better control over sodium content.

2. Potassium Regulation:
    1. Monitor potassium intake, as elevated levels can affect heart function.

2. Limit high-potassium fruits (bananas, oranges, melons) and vegetables (potatoes, tomatoes, spinach).
3. Choose low-potassium alternatives like apples, berries, and green beans.
4. Ensure proper cooking techniques, such as leaching or soaking vegetables to reduce potassium.

3. Phosphorus Control:
   1. Restrict high-phosphorus foods, especially processed and fast foods.
   2. Limit dairy products and choose phosphorus binders as recommended by the healthcare team.
   3. Select lean protein sources to reduce phosphorus intake.
   4. Be cautious with nuts, seeds, and colas, which are high in phosphorus.

4. Protein Moderation:
   1. Consume moderate amounts of high-quality protein to minimize kidney workload.
   2. Choose lean protein sources like poultry, fish, eggs, and plant-based proteins.
   3. Monitor protein intake to avoid excessive levels that may strain the kidneys.
   4. Consider consulting a dietitian for personalized protein recommendations.

 KIDNEY DISEASE DIET FOODS CHART FOR SENIORS ON STAGE 3

5. Fluid Management:
   1. Monitor fluid intake based on individual needs and recommendations.
   2. Adjust fluid intake based on urine output, climate, and activity level.
   3. Be mindful of hidden fluids in foods (soups, fruits, gelatin).
   4. Limit caffeine and alcohol, as they can contribute to fluid loss.

6. Individualized Caloric Intake:
   1. Adjust caloric intake based on individual factors such as age, weight, and physical activity.
   2. Ensure an appropriate balance of macronutrients (carbohydrates, proteins, fats) within recommended levels.
   3. Consult with a dietitian to create a personalized meal plan.

7. Monitor Blood Sugar Levels:
   1. If diabetic, manage blood sugar levels through a balanced diet, medication, and regular monitoring.
   2. Control intake of high-sugar foods and beverages.

8. Limit Phosphorus Additives:
   1. Be aware of phosphorus additives in processed foods; read labels carefully.

2. Choose whole, unprocessed foods whenever possible.

9. Regular Monitoring:
   1. Regularly monitor blood pressure, kidney function, and relevant laboratory values.
   2. Adjust the diet based on healthcare professional recommendations and changes in health status.

10. Consult with Healthcare Professionals:
- Collaborate closely with a healthcare team, including a nephrologist and registered dietitian.
- Keep open communication about dietary changes, symptoms, and overall health.

Kidney friendly meal plan tips for seniors with stage 3 CKD

Meal planning for seniors with Stage 3 Chronic Kidney Disease (CKD) involves careful consideration of nutrient intake, especially regarding sodium, potassium, phosphorus, protein, and fluid. Here are detailed kidney-friendly meal planning tips for seniors with Stage 3 CKD:

1. Work with a Dietitian:
Consult a registered dietitian who specializes in renal nutrition. They can provide personalized

guidance based on the individual's health status, preferences, and specific dietary needs.

2. Portion Control:
Pay attention to portion sizes to avoid overconsumption of nutrients like phosphorus and protein. Use smaller plates to help control portions.

3. Monitor Protein Intake:
   1. Choose high-quality, lean protein sources such as poultry, fish, eggs, and plant-based proteins like beans and lentils.
   2. Limit red meat and processed meats, as they are higher in phosphorus.

4. Control Phosphorus Intake:
   1. Choose low-phosphorus foods, especially when it comes to dairy products, nuts, seeds, and processed foods.
   2. Use phosphorus binders as prescribed by healthcare professionals.

5. Choose Low-Potassium Fruits and Vegetables:
   1. Opt for fruits and vegetables lower in potassium, such as apples, berries, and green beans.
   2. Cook vegetables in water to reduce potassium content.

6. Manage Sodium Intake:
   1. Limit processed and packaged foods, as they often contain high levels of sodium.
   2. Use herbs, spices, and lemon juice for flavor instead of salt.
   3. Rinse canned vegetables and beans to reduce sodium content.

7. Fluid Management:
   1. Monitor fluid intake based on individual needs, considering factors like urine output, climate, and activity level.
   2. Distribute fluid intake throughout the day to avoid excessive fluid at one time.

8. Plan Balanced Meals:
   1. Aim for a well-balanced diet with a mix of carbohydrates, proteins, and healthy fats.
   2. Include a variety of vegetables to provide essential vitamins and minerals.

9. Limit High-Sugar Foods:
   1. Control blood sugar levels by limiting high-sugar foods and beverages.
   2. Choose whole, unprocessed grains to minimize phosphorus intake.

10. Keep a Food Diary:
- Track daily food intake to monitor adherence to dietary recommendations and identify potential issues.

11. Cooking Techniques:
- Choose cooking methods that retain nutrients without adding unnecessary ones. Steaming, baking, and grilling are good options.
- Leach high-potassium vegetables by soaking them in water before cooking.

12. Individualized Meal Plans:
- Tailor meal plans to individual preferences, cultural considerations, and dietary restrictions.
- Adjust meal plans based on lab results and any changes in health status.

13. Educate Caregivers:
- Ensure that caregivers and family members are educated about the specific dietary restrictions and requirements.

14. Medication Adherence:
- Take prescribed medications as directed by healthcare professionals, including phosphorus binders.

15. Regular Monitoring:
- Stay proactive with regular check-ups, monitoring blood pressure, and adjusting the

meal plan based on healthcare professional recommendations.

16. Enjoying Special Occasions:
- Find kidney-friendly alternatives during special occasions to maintain social connections without compromising dietary restrictions.

17. Be Mindful of Hidden Phosphorus and Potassium:
- Read food labels carefully to identify hidden phosphorus and potassium additives in processed foods.

LIST OF FOODS TO ENJOY WHILE ON FRIENDLY KIDNEY DIET

Fruits

Apples:
Sodium: 0mg
Calories (per medium apple): 95
Other Nutrients: Dietary fiber (4g), Vitamin C (14% DV), Potassium (195mg)

Bananas:
Sodium: 1mg
Calories (per medium banana): 105
Other Nutrients: Dietary fiber (3g), Vitamin C (10% DV), Potassium (422mg)

Berries (Strawberries, Blueberries, Raspberries):
Sodium: 1-2mg (per cup)
Calories (per cup): 50-85
Other Nutrients: Dietary fiber, Vitamin C, Antioxidants

Grapes:
Sodium: 2mg
Calories (per cup): 104
Other Nutrients: Dietary fiber (1g), Vitamin C (5% DV), Potassium (288mg)

Watermelon:
Sodium: 2mg
Calories (per cup, diced): 46
Other Nutrients: Vitamin C (13% DV), Potassium (170mg)

Cucumbers:
Sodium: 2mg
Calories (per cup, sliced): 16
Other Nutrients: Vitamin K (14% DV), Vitamin C (4% DV)

Pineapple:
Sodium: 1mg
Calories (per cup, chunks): 83
Other Nutrients: Dietary fiber (2g), Vitamin C (79% DV)

Oranges:
Sodium: 0mg
Calories (per medium orange): 62
Other Nutrients: Dietary fiber (3g), Vitamin C (70% DV), Potassium (237mg)

Kiwi:
Sodium: 3mg
Calories (per medium kiwi): 61
Other Nutrients: Dietary fiber (3g), Vitamin C (92% DV), Potassium (273mg)

Mango:
Sodium: 1mg
Calories (per cup, sliced): 107
Other Nutrients: Vitamin C (60% DV), Vitamin A (10% DV)

Pears:
Sodium: 0mg
Calories (per medium pear): 101
Other Nutrients: Dietary fiber (5g), Vitamin C (7% DV), Potassium (195mg)

Apricots:
Sodium: 1mg
Calories (per apricot): 17
Other Nutrients: Vitamin A (34% DV), Vitamin C (8% DV)

Plums:
Sodium: 0mg
Calories (per plum): 30
Other Nutrients: Dietary fiber (1g), Vitamin C
(10% DV), Vitamin K (5% DV)

Cantaloupe:
Sodium: 29mg
Calories (per cup, cubes): 54
Other Nutrients: Vitamin C (68% DV), Vitamin
A (54% DV)

Cherries:
Sodium: 0mg
Calories (per cup): 87
Other Nutrients: Dietary fiber (3g), Vitamin C
(16% DV)

Cranberries:
Sodium: 2mg
Calories (per cup): 51
Other Nutrients: Dietary fiber (4g), Vitamin C
(24% DV)

Grapefruit:
Sodium: 0mg
Calories (per half): 52
Other Nutrients: Dietary fiber (2g), Vitamin C
(64% DV), Potassium (166mg)

Raisins:
Sodium: 2mg
Calories (per small box, about 43g): 129
Other Nutrients: Dietary fiber (1g), Iron (1mg)

Blackberries:
Sodium: 1mg
Calories (per cup): 62
Other Nutrients: Dietary fiber (8g), Vitamin C (50% DV)

Peaches:
Sodium: 0mg
Calories (per medium peach): 58
Other Nutrients: Dietary fiber (2g), Vitamin C (10% DV)

Vegetables

Cucumbers:
Sodium: 2mg
Calories (per cup, sliced): 16
Other Nutrients: Vitamin K (14% DV), Vitamin C (4% DV)

Carrots:
Sodium: 42mg
Calories (per cup, sliced): 50
Other Nutrients: Vitamin A (428% DV), Vitamin K (13% DV), Fiber (3.6g)

Bell Peppers (Green, Red, Yellow):
Sodium: 3mg
Calories (per cup, sliced): 46
Other Nutrients: Vitamin C (200% DV), Vitamin
A (93% DV)

Broccoli:
Sodium: 30mg
Calories (per cup, chopped): 55
Other Nutrients: Vitamin C (135% DV), Vitamin
K (115% DV), Fiber (3.7g)

Spinach:
Sodium: 24mg
Calories (per cup, raw): 7
Other Nutrients: Vitamin A (56% DV), Vitamin
K (47% DV), Iron (0.8mg)

Cabbage:
Sodium: 12mg
Calories (per cup, chopped): 22
Other Nutrients: Vitamin C (54% DV), Vitamin
K (85% DV), Fiber (2.2g)

Zucchini:
Sodium: 8mg
Calories (per cup, sliced): 20
Other Nutrients: Vitamin C (21% DV), Vitamin
B6 (10% DV), Fiber (1.2g)

Cauliflower:
Sodium: 30mg
Calories (per cup, chopped): 27
Other Nutrients: Vitamin C (77% DV), Vitamin K (20% DV), Fiber (2.5g)

Asparagus:
Sodium: 2mg
Calories (per cup, chopped): 27
Other Nutrients: Vitamin K (55% DV), Folate (34% DV), Fiber (2.8g)

Brussels Sprouts:
Sodium: 16mg
Calories (per cup, cooked): 56
Other Nutrients: Vitamin C (129% DV), Vitamin K (137% DV), Fiber (4g)

Kale:
Sodium: 23mg
Calories (per cup, chopped): 33
Other Nutrients: Vitamin A (206% DV), Vitamin K (684% DV), Fiber (2.6g)

Eggplant:
Sodium: 2mg
Calories (per cup, cubed): 20
Other Nutrients: Fiber (2.5g), Folate (6% DV)

Green Beans:
Sodium: 6mg
Calories (per cup, cooked): 44
Other Nutrients: Vitamin C (27% DV), Vitamin K (14% DV), Fiber (4g)

Celery:
Sodium: 32mg
Calories (per cup, chopped): 16
Other Nutrients: Vitamin K (30% DV), Fiber (1.6g)

Onions:
Sodium: 2mg
Calories (per medium onion): 44
Other Nutrients: Vitamin C (12% DV), Fiber (3.1g)

Tomatoes:
Sodium: 9mg
Calories (per medium tomato): 22
Other Nutrients: Vitamin C (28% DV), Vitamin A (20% DV)

Mushrooms:
Sodium: 5mg
Calories (per cup, sliced): 15
Other Nutrients: Vitamin D (2% DV), Selenium (8% DV)

Sweet Potatoes:
Sodium: 12mg
Calories (per medium sweet potato): 103
Other Nutrients: Vitamin A (438% DV), Vitamin

Lettuce (Iceberg, Romaine):
Sodium: 5mg
Calories (per cup, shredded): 5
Other Nutrients: Vitamin A (31% DV), Vitamin
K (89% DV)

Beets:
Sodium: 65mg
Calories (per cup, cooked): 75
Other Nutrients: Vitamin C (8% DV), Fiber
(3.4g)

Lean protein

Chicken Breast (Skinless, Grilled):
Sodium: 74mg (per 3-ounce serving)
Calories: 165
Other Nutrients: Protein (31g), Iron (1mg),
Vitamin B6 (0.5mg)

Turkey (Lean Ground, Cooked):
Sodium: 60mg (per 3-ounce serving)
Calories: 193
Other Nutrients: Protein (19g), Iron (2.4mg)

Fish (Salmon, Baked or Grilled):
Sodium: 50mg (per 3-ounce serving)
Calories: 206
Other Nutrients: Protein (22g), Omega-3 Fatty Acids (1.1g), Vitamin D (570 IU)

Tuna (Canned in Water):
Sodium: 230mg (per 3-ounce serving)
Calories: 99
Other Nutrients: Protein (22g), Omega-3 Fatty Acids (0.2g)

Cod (Baked or Grilled):
Sodium: 74mg (per 3-ounce serving)
Calories: 89
Other Nutrients: Protein (19g), Vitamin B12 (1.1mcg), Selenium (20mcg)

Shrimp (Boiled or Grilled):
Sodium: 120mg (per 3-ounce serving)
Calories: 84
Other Nutrients: Protein (18g), Selenium (31mcg)

Eggs:
Sodium: 70mg (per large egg)
Calories: 72
Other Nutrients: Protein (6g), Vitamin B12 (0.6mcg), Choline (147mg)

Lean Beef (Top Sirloin, Grilled):
Sodium: 55mg (per 3-ounce serving)
Calories: 159
Other Nutrients: Protein (26g), Iron (2.6mg), Zinc (5.4mg)

Pork Tenderloin (Roasted):
Sodium: 50mg (per 3-ounce serving)
Calories: 143
Other Nutrients: Protein (24g), Thiamine (0.8mg), Selenium (24mcg)

Veal (Lean, Roasted):
Sodium: 72mg (per 3-ounce serving)
Calories: 135
Other Nutrients: Protein (24g), Iron (1.5mg), Zinc (2.7mg)

Chicken Thigh (Skinless, Grilled):
Sodium: 77mg (per 3-ounce serving)
Calories: 209
Other Nutrients: Protein (26g), Iron (1.1mg)

Lamb (Leg, Roasted):
Sodium: 76mg (per 3-ounce serving)
Calories: 172
Other Nutrients: Protein (23g), Iron (1.9mg), Vitamin B12 (2.6mcg)

Lean Ground Beef (90% Lean, Cooked):
Sodium: 72mg (per 3-ounce serving)
Calories: 184
Other Nutrients: Protein (22g), Iron (2.1mg),
Zinc (6.2mg)

Chicken Drumstick (Skinless, Roasted):
Sodium: 81mg (per 3-ounce serving)
Calories: 174
Other Nutrients: Protein (20g), Iron (1.1mg)

Cottage Cheese (Low-Fat):
Sodium: 459mg (per cup)
Calories: 206
Other Nutrients: Protein (28g), Calcium (220mg)

Greek Yogurt (Non-fat):
Sodium: 59mg (per 6-ounce container)
Calories: 100
Other Nutrients: Protein (15g), Calcium (183mg)

Soybeans (Boiled):
Sodium: 2mg (per half-cup)
Calories: 127
Other Nutrients: Protein (11g), Fiber (5g), Iron
(1.8mg)

Tofu (Firm):
Sodium: 8mg (per 3-ounce serving)
Calories: 70
Other Nutrients: Protein (8g), Calcium (350mg),
Iron (2mg)

Chicken Liver (Pan-Fried):
Sodium: 58mg (per 3-ounce serving)
Calories: 174
Other Nutrients: Protein (23g), Iron (13.6mg),
Vitamin A (26,000 IU)

Chicken Wings (Skinless, Grilled):
Sodium: 71mg (per 3-ounce serving)
Calories: 203
Other Nutrients: Protein (24g), Iron (1.1mg)

Catfish (Baked or Grilled):
Sodium: 59mg (per 3-ounce serving)
Calories: 105
Other Nutrients: Protein (20g), Vitamin B12
(2.4mcg)

Grains and Starches

Brown Rice (Cooked):
Sodium: 5mg (per cup)
Calories: 215
Other Nutrients: Fiber (3.5g), B Vitamins

Quinoa (Cooked):
Sodium: 13mg (per cup)
Calories: 222
Other Nutrients: Protein (8g), Fiber (5g), Iron (2.8mg)

Oats (Rolled or Steel-Cut, Cooked):
Sodium: 2mg (per cup)
Calories: 150
Other Nutrients: Fiber (4g), Iron (1.7mg)

Buckwheat (Cooked):
Sodium: 1mg (per cup)
Calories: 154
Other Nutrients: Protein (6g), Fiber (4.5g), Magnesium (86mg)

Millet (Cooked):
Sodium: 2mg (per cup)
Calories: 207
Other Nutrients: Protein (6g), Fiber (2.3g), Magnesium (76mg)

Barley (Cooked):
Sodium: 5mg (per cup)
Calories: 193
Other Nutrients: Fiber (6g), Iron (1.6mg)

Whole Wheat Pasta (Cooked):
Sodium: 3mg (per cup)
Calories: 174
Other Nutrients: Protein (7.5g), Fiber (6.3g)

Sweet Potatoes (Baked):
Sodium: 12mg (per medium-sized potato)
Calories: 103
Other Nutrients: Fiber (3.8g), Vitamin A (438% DV), Vitamin C (24% DV)

Butternut Squash (Baked):
Sodium: 6mg (per cup, cubes)
Calories: 82
Other Nutrients: Fiber (2.8g), Vitamin A (438% DV), Vitamin C (23% DV)

Wild Rice (Cooked):
Sodium: 5mg (per cup)
Calories: 166
Other Nutrients: Fiber (3g), Protein (6.5g)

Couscous (Cooked, Whole Wheat):
Sodium: 4mg (per cup)
Calories: 176
Other Nutrients: Protein (6g), Fiber (5.2g)

Basmati Rice (Cooked):
Sodium: 1mg (per cup)
Calories: 205
Other Nutrients: Fiber (1.6g)

Spaghetti Squash (Baked):
Sodium: 17mg (per cup)
Calories: 42
Other Nutrients: Fiber (2.2g), Vitamin C (9% DV)

Whole Wheat Bread:
Sodium: 134mg (per slice)
Calories: 69
Other Nutrients: Fiber (1.9g)

Rye Bread:
Sodium: 183mg (per slice)
Calories: 83
Other Nutrients: Fiber (1.9g)

Whole Grain Crackers:
Sodium: 135mg (per 6 crackers)
Calories: 120
Other Nutrients: Fiber (2g)

Corn Tortillas:
Sodium: 3mg (per medium-sized tortilla)
Calories: 52
Other Nutrients: Fiber (0.8g)

Brown Lentils (Cooked):
Sodium: 1mg (per cup)
Calories: 230
Other Nutrients: Protein (18g), Fiber (16g), Iron (6.6mg)

Chickpeas (Canned):
Sodium: 2mg (per cup)
Calories: 269
Other Nutrients: Protein (15g), Fiber (13g), Iron (4.7mg)

Black Beans (Canned):
Sodium: 2mg (per cup)
Calories: 227
Other Nutrients: Protein (15g), Fiber (15g), Iron (3.6mg)

Dairy and Dairy Alternatives

Skim Milk:
Sodium: 98mg (per cup)
Calories: 83
Other Nutrients: Calcium (299mg), Vitamin D (125 IU)

Low-Fat Yogurt:
Sodium: 87mg (per 6-ounce container)
Calories: 154
Other Nutrients: Protein (14g), Calcium (448mg)

Cottage Cheese (Low-Fat):
Sodium: 459mg (per cup)
Calories: 206
Other Nutrients: Protein (28g), Calcium (220mg)

Greek Yogurt (Non-fat):
Sodium: 59mg (per 6-ounce container)
Calories: 100
Other Nutrients: Protein (15g), Calcium (183mg)

Ricotta Cheese (Part-Skim):
Sodium: 42mg (per 1/2 cup)
Calories: 337
Other Nutrients: Protein (14g), Calcium (337mg)

String Cheese (Part-Skim):
Sodium: 174mg (per stick)
Calories: 80
Other Nutrients: Protein (7g), Calcium (183mg)

Buttermilk:
Sodium: 260mg (per cup)
Calories: 98
Other Nutrients: Calcium (284mg), Vitamin D (115 IU)

Swiss Cheese (Low-Sodium):
Sodium: Varies (check label)
Calories: Varies
Other Nutrients: Protein, Calcium

Mozzarella Cheese (Part-Skim):
Sodium: 176mg (per 1 ounce)
Calories: 72
Other Nutrients: Protein (7g), Calcium (183mg)

Cheddar Cheese (Low-Sodium):
Sodium: Varies (check label)
Calories: Varies
Other Nutrients: Protein, Calcium

Cream Cheese (Low-Sodium):
Sodium: Varies (check label)
Calories: Varies
Other Nutrients: Protein, Calcium

Sour Cream (Reduced-Fat):
Sodium: 24mg (per tablespoon)
Calories: 16
Other Nutrients: Calcium (14mg)

Parmesan Cheese (Grated):
Sodium: 76mg (per tablespoon)
Calories: 21
Other Nutrients: Protein (2g), Calcium (83mg)

Low-Fat Chocolate Milk:
Sodium: 107mg (per cup)
Calories: 158
Other Nutrients: Calcium (284mg), Vitamin D (115 IU)

Almond Milk (Unsweetened):
Sodium: 150mg (per cup)
Calories: 13
Other Nutrients: Calcium (516mg), Vitamin D (120 IU)

Coconut Milk (Unsweetened):
Sodium: 15mg (per cup)
Calories: 50
Other Nutrients: Calcium (460mg), Vitamin D (0 IU)

Soy Milk (Unsweetened):
Sodium: 72mg (per cup)
Calories: 80
Other Nutrients: Protein (7g), Calcium (299mg)

Oat Milk (Unsweetened):
Sodium: 95mg (per cup)
Calories: 80
Other Nutrients: Calcium (350mg), Vitamin D (120 IU)

Rice Milk (Unsweetened):
Sodium: 10mg (per cup)
Calories: 120
Other Nutrients: Calcium (283mg), Vitamin D (120 IU)

Hemp Milk (Unsweetened):
Sodium: 0mg (per cup)
Calories: 70
Other Nutrients: Calcium (283mg), Vitamin D (120 IU)

Kefir (Plain):
Sodium: 85mg (per cup)
Calories: 100
Other Nutrients: Protein (10g), Calcium (336mg)

Goat Cheese (Soft):
Sodium: 114mg (per ounce)
Calories: 103
Other Nutrients: Protein (6g), Calcium (68mg)

Blue Cheese (Low-Sodium):
Sodium: Varies (check label)
Calories: Varies
Other Nutrients: Protein, Calcium

Herbs and Spices

Basil (Fresh):
Sodium: 0mg (per tablespoon)
Calories: 1
Other Nutrients: Vitamin A (98% DV), Vitamin K (36% DV)

Cilantro (Fresh):
Sodium: 1mg (per tablespoon)
Calories: 0
Other Nutrients: Vitamin A (34% DV), Vitamin K (16% DV)

Parsley (Fresh):
Sodium: 1mg (per tablespoon)
Calories: 1
Other Nutrients: Vitamin A (54% DV), Vitamin C (22% DV)

Dill (Fresh):
Sodium: 1mg (per tablespoon)
Calories: 1
Other Nutrients: Vitamin A (29% DV), Vitamin C (20% DV)

Chives (Fresh):
Sodium: 1mg (per tablespoon)
Calories: 1
Other Nutrients: Vitamin A (22% DV), Vitamin C (10% DV)

Mint (Fresh):
Sodium: 0mg (per tablespoon)
Calories: 1
Other Nutrients: Vitamin A (12% DV), Vitamin C (7% DV)

Rosemary (Dried):
Sodium: 1mg (per teaspoon)
Calories: 2
Other Nutrients: Iron (0.1mg), Calcium (8mg)

Thyme (Dried):
Sodium: 1mg (per teaspoon)
Calories: 3
Other Nutrients: Iron (0.1mg), Vitamin C (1mg)

 KIDNEY DISEASE DIET FOODS CHART FOR SENIORS ON STAGE 3

Oregano (Dried):
Sodium: 1mg (per teaspoon)
Calories: 3
Other Nutrients: Iron (0.1mg), Calcium (29mg)

Sage (Dried):
Sodium: 1mg (per teaspoon)
Calories: 3
Other Nutrients: Vitamin K (10% DV), Iron (0.3mg)

Bay Leaves (Dried):
Sodium: 1mg (per leaf)
Calories: 2
Other Nutrients: Iron (0.2mg), Vitamin A (3% DV)

Cayenne Pepper (Ground):
Sodium: 1mg (per teaspoon)
Calories: 6
Other Nutrients: Vitamin A (44% DV), Vitamin C (3% DV)

Black Pepper (Ground):
Sodium: 0mg (per teaspoon)
Calories: 5
Other Nutrients: Manganese (0.1mg), Vitamin K (2% DV)

Cumin (Ground):
Sodium: 1mg (per teaspoon)
Calories: 8
Other Nutrients: Iron (1.4mg), Vitamin C (1mg)

Coriander (Ground):
Sodium: 2mg (per teaspoon)
Calories: 5
Other Nutrients: Iron (0.4mg), Vitamin C (1mg)

Paprika (Ground):
Sodium: 1mg (per teaspoon)
Calories: 6
Other Nutrients: Vitamin A (897 IU), Vitamin C (1mg)

Turmeric (Ground):
Sodium: 2mg (per teaspoon)
Calories: 8
Other Nutrients: Iron (1.8mg), Vitamin C (1mg)

Ginger (Ground):
Sodium: 1mg (per teaspoon)
Calories: 6
Other Nutrients: Manganese (0.1mg), Vitamin C (1mg)

Garlic Powder:
Sodium: 1mg (per teaspoon)
Calories: 10
Other Nutrients: Vitamin C (2mg), Calcium (30mg)

Onion Powder:
Sodium: 1mg (per teaspoon)
Calories: 8
Other Nutrients: Vitamin C (2mg), Calcium (16mg)

Cinnamon (Ground):
Sodium: 0mg (per teaspoon)
Calories: 6
Other Nutrients: Calcium (26mg), Iron (0.5mg)

Nutmeg (Ground):
Sodium: 0mg (per teaspoon)
Calories: 12
Other Nutrients: Manganese (0.3mg), Iron (0.2mg)

Cloves (Ground):
Sodium: 1mg (per teaspoon)
Calories: 6
Other Nutrients: Manganese (0.1mg), Vitamin C (1mg)

Snacks

1. Fresh Fruit Salad:
Sodium: 1mg (per cup)
Calories: 60
Other Nutrients: Fiber, Vitamins, Antioxidants

2. Raw Vegetable Sticks (Carrots, Cucumbers)
with Hummus:
Sodium: Varies (check hummus label)
Calories: Varies
Other Nutrients: Fiber, Vitamins, Protein

3. Air-Popped Popcorn (Unsalted):
Sodium: 1mg (per cup)
Calories: 31
Other Nutrients: Fiber, Whole Grains

4. Rice Cakes with Almond Butter:
Sodium: Varies (check almond butter label)
Calories: Varies
Other Nutrients: Protein, Healthy Fats

5. Greek Yogurt with Fresh Berries:
Sodium: Varies (check yogurt label)
Calories: Varies
Other Nutrients: Protein, Calcium, Probiotics

6. Apple Slices with Peanut Butter:
Sodium: 1mg (per tablespoon of unsalted peanut butter)
Calories: Varies
Other Nutrients: Fiber, Protein

7. Nuts (Almonds, Walnuts, or Pistachios):
Sodium: Varies
Calories: Varies
Other Nutrients: Healthy Fats, Protein

8. Cottage Cheese with Pineapple Chunks:
Sodium: Varies (check cottage cheese label)
Calories: Varies
Other Nutrients: Protein, Calcium

9. Banana with Almond or Sunflower Seed Butter:
Sodium: Varies (check nut or seed butter label)
Calories: Varies
Other Nutrients: Fiber, Protein, Healthy Fats

10. Veggie Chips (Homemade or Low-Sodium Store-Bought):
- Sodium: Varies (check label)
- Calories: Varies
- Other Nutrients: Fiber, Vitamins

11. Hard-Boiled Eggs:
- Sodium: 70mg (per large egg)
- Calories: 68
- Other Nutrients: Protein, Vitamins

12. Fresh Berries (Strawberries, Blueberries) with Whipped Cream:
- Sodium: Varies (check whipped cream label)
- Calories: Varies
- Other Nutrients: Fiber, Antioxidants

13. Dark Chocolate (Low-Sodium):
- Sodium: Varies (check label)
- Calories: Varies
- Other Nutrients: Antioxidants

14. Celery Sticks with Cream Cheese (Low-Sodium):
- Sodium: Varies (check cream cheese label)
- Calories: Varies
- Other Nutrients: Fiber, Calcium

15. Trail Mix (Nuts, Seeds, Dried Fruits, Unsweetened):
- Sodium: Varies (check label)
- Calories: Varies
- Other Nutrients: Healthy Fats, Fiber, Protein

16. Fresh Peach or Plum Slices:
- Sodium: 0mg (per fruit)
- Calories: Varies

 KIDNEY DISEASE DIET FOODS CHART FOR SENIORS ON STAGE 3

- Other Nutrients: Fiber, Vitamins

17. Yogurt Parfait with Granola (Low-Sodium):
- Sodium: Varies (check granola and yogurt labels)
- Calories: Varies
- Other Nutrients: Protein, Calcium, Fiber

18. Roasted Chickpeas (Unsalted):
- Sodium: 2mg (per 1/2 cup)
- Calories: 134
- Other Nutrients: Protein, Fiber

19. Low-Sodium Cheese Cubes:
- Sodium: Varies (check label)
- Calories: Varies
- Other Nutrients: Protein, Calcium

20. Sliced Watermelon:
- Sodium: 2mg (per cup)
- Calories: 46
- Other Nutrients: Hydration, Vitamins

Beverages

1. Water:
Sodium: 0mg (per 8 ounces)
Calories: 0
Other Nutrients: Hydration

2. Herbal Tea (Unsweetened):
Sodium: 0mg (per 8 ounces)
Calories: 0
Other Nutrients: Antioxidants

3. Green Tea (Unsweetened):
Sodium: 0mg (per 8 ounces)
Calories: 0
Other Nutrients: Catechins, Antioxidants

4. Black Tea (Unsweetened):
Sodium: 0mg (per 8 ounces)
Calories: 2
Other Nutrients: Caffeine, Antioxidants

5. Lemonade (Homemade, Low-Sugar):
Sodium: 1mg (per cup)
Calories: 50
Other Nutrients: Vitamin C

6. Coconut Water (Unsweetened):
Sodium: 24mg (per cup)
Calories: 46
Other Nutrients: Electrolytes

7. Freshly Squeezed Orange Juice (Diluted with Water):
Sodium: 1mg (per cup)
Calories: 80
Other Nutrients: Vitamin C

8. Cranberry Juice (100% Unsweetened):
Sodium: 2mg (per cup)
Calories: 46
Other Nutrients: Antioxidants

9. Almond Milk (Unsweetened):
Sodium: 150mg (per cup)
Calories: 13
Other Nutrients: Calcium, Vitamin D

10. Soy Milk (Unsweetened):
- Sodium: 72mg (per cup)
- Calories: 80
- Other Nutrients: Protein, Calcium

11. Rice Milk (Unsweetened):
- Sodium: 10mg (per cup)
- Calories: 120
- Other Nutrients: Calcium, Vitamin D

12. Oat Milk (Unsweetened):
- Sodium: 95mg (per cup)
- Calories: 80
- Other Nutrients: Fiber, Calcium

13. Carrot Juice (Unsweetened):
- Sodium: 77mg (per cup)
- Calories: 94
- Other Nutrients: Vitamin A, Vitamin K

14. Tomato Juice (Low-Sodium):
- Sodium: Varies (check label)
- Calories: Varies
- Other Nutrients: Lycopene, Vitamins

15. Apple Cider Vinegar Drink (Diluted with Water):
- Sodium: 2mg (per tablespoon)
- Calories: 1
- Other Nutrients: Acetic Acid

16. Iced Herbal Infusions (Mint, Hibiscus):
- Sodium: 0mg (per 8 ounces)
- Calories: 0
- Other Nutrients: Hydration, Antioxidants

17. Sparkling Water (Unsweetened):
- Sodium: 0mg (per 8 ounces)
- Calories: 0
- Other Nutrients: Hydration

18. Ginger Tea (Unsweetened):
- Sodium: 0mg (per 8 ounces)
- Calories: 0
- Other Nutrients: Anti-Inflammatory

 KIDNEY DISEASE DIET FOODS CHART FOR SENIORS ON STAGE 3

19. Buttermilk (Low-Fat):
- Sodium: 260mg (per cup)
- Calories: 98
- Other Nutrients: Calcium, Vitamin D

20. Pineapple Juice (100% Unsweetened):
- Sodium: 2mg (per cup)
- Calories: 132
- Other Nutrients: Vitamin C, Manganese

21. Peach Iced Tea (Unsweetened):
- Sodium: 0mg (per 8 ounces)
- Calories: 0
- Other Nutrients: Hydration, Antioxidants

22. Beet Juice (Unsweetened):
- Sodium: 75mg (per cup)
- Calories: 70
- Other Nutrients: Nitrates, Iron

Canned Goods

1. Low-Sodium Canned Beans (Black Beans, Kidney Beans, Chickpeas):
Sodium: 5mg (per 1/2 cup)
Calories: 110
Other Nutrients: Fiber, Protein

2. No-Salt-Added Canned Tomatoes:
Sodium: 10mg (per 1/2 cup)
Calories: 20
Other Nutrients: Vitamin C, Lycopene

3. Low-Sodium Canned Corn:
Sodium: 10mg (per 1/2 cup)
Calories: 60
Other Nutrients: Fiber, Vitamin C

4. Low-Sodium Canned Peas:
Sodium: 4mg (per 1/2 cup)
Calories: 60
Other Nutrients: Fiber, Protein

5. Low-Sodium Canned Tuna (in water):
Sodium: 180mg (per 3-ounce serving)
Calories: 100
Other Nutrients: Protein, Omega-3 Fatty Acids

6. Low-Sodium Canned Salmon (Wild-caught, in water):
Sodium: 50mg (per 3-ounce serving)
Calories: 120
Other Nutrients: Protein, Omega-3 Fatty Acids

7. Low-Sodium Canned Chicken Breast:
Sodium: 150mg (per 2-ounce serving)
Calories: 60
Other Nutrients: Protein

8. Low-Sodium Canned Green Beans:
Sodium: 5mg (per 1/2 cup)
Calories: 20
Other Nutrients: Fiber, Vitamin C

9. Low-Sodium Canned Carrots:
Sodium: 25mg (per 1/2 cup)
Calories: 30
Other Nutrients: Fiber, Vitamin A

10. Low-Sodium Canned Beets:
- Sodium: 35mg (per 1/2 cup)
- Calories: 37
- Other Nutrients: Fiber, Folate

11. Low-Sodium Canned Pineapple Chunks (in juice):
- Sodium: 0mg (per 1/2 cup)
- Calories: 60
- Other Nutrients: Vitamin C, Manganese

12. Low-Sodium Canned Mandarin Oranges (in juice):
- Sodium: 0mg (per 1/2 cup)
- Calories: 50
- Other Nutrients: Vitamin C

13. Low-Sodium Canned Mixed Vegetables:
- Sodium: 40mg (per 1/2 cup)
- Calories: 60
- Other Nutrients: Fiber, Vitamins

14. Low-Sodium Canned Peaches (in juice):
- Sodium: 0mg (per 1/2 cup)
- Calories: 50
- Other Nutrients: Vitamin C

15. Low-Sodium Canned Pears (in juice):
- Sodium: 0mg (per 1/2 cup)
- Calories: 50
- Other Nutrients: Fiber, Vitamin C

16. Low-Sodium Canned Artichoke Hearts:
- Sodium: 70mg (per 1/2 cup)
- Calories: 30
- Other Nutrients: Fiber

17. Low-Sodium Canned Asparagus:
- Sodium: 20mg (per 1/2 cup)
- Calories: 20
- Other Nutrients: Fiber, Folate

18. Low-Sodium Canned Spinach:
- Sodium: 30mg (per 1/2 cup)
- Calories: 15
- Other Nutrients: Iron, Vitamin A

19. Low-Sodium Canned Pumpkin:
- Sodium: 5mg (per 1/2 cup)
- Calories: 25
- Other Nutrients: Fiber, Vitamin A

20. Low-Sodium Canned Sweet Potatoes:
- Sodium: 30mg (per 1/2 cup)
- Calories: 90
- Other Nutrients: Fiber, Vitamin A

21. Low-Sodium Canned Lentils:
- Sodium: 10mg (per 1/2 cup)
- Calories: 120
- Other Nutrients: Protein, Fiber

22. Low-Sodium Canned Black-Eyed Peas:
- Sodium: 10mg (per 1/2 cup)
- Calories: 70
- Other Nutrients: Protein, Fiber

23. Low-Sodium Canned Green Peas:
- Sodium: 5mg (per 1/2 cup)
- Calories: 60
- Other Nutrients: Fiber, Protein

Low-Potassium Fruits

Apples (1 medium):
Potassium: 195mg
Calories: 95
Other Nutrients: Fiber, Vitamin C

Berries (Strawberries, Blueberries, Raspberries -1 cup):
Potassium: 150-250mg
Calories: 50-85
Other Nutrients: Fiber, Antioxidants, Vitamin C

Pineapple (1/2 cup):
Potassium: 120mg
Calories: 41
Other Nutrients: Vitamin C, Manganese

Peaches (1 medium):
Potassium: 200mg
Calories: 60
Other Nutrients: Vitamin A, Vitamin C

Pears (1 medium):
Potassium: 200mg
Calories: 101
Other Nutrients: Fiber, Vitamin C

Plums (1 medium):
Potassium: 100mg
Calories: 30
Other Nutrients: Fiber, Vitamin C

Grapes (1 cup):
Potassium: 288mg
Calories: 104
Other Nutrients: Antioxidants, Vitamin K

Watermelon (1 cup):
Potassium: 170mg
Calories: 46
Other Nutrients: Hydration, Vitamin A, Vitamin C

Cantaloupe (1/2 cup):
Potassium: 215mg
Calories: 27
Other Nutrients: Vitamin A, Vitamin C

Honeydew Melon (1/2 cup):
Potassium: 228mg
Calories: 31
Other Nutrients: Vitamin C

Apricots (2 medium):
Potassium: 116mg
Calories: 34
Other Nutrients: Vitamin A, Vitamin C

Cranberries (1 cup, unsweetened):
Potassium: 90mg
Calories: 46
Other Nutrients: Antioxidants, Vitamin C

Kiwi (1 medium):
Potassium: 215mg
Calories: 61
Other Nutrients: Fiber, Vitamin C, Vitamin K

Oranges (1 medium):
Potassium: 237mg
Calories: 62
Other Nutrients: Vitamin C, Fiber

Mango (1/2 cup, sliced):
Potassium: 118mg
Calories: 54
Other Nutrients: Vitamin A, Vitamin C

Nectarines (1 medium):
Potassium: 234mg
Calories: 62
Other Nutrients: Vitamin A, Vitamin C

Cherries (1 cup):
Potassium: 260mg
Calories: 97
Other Nutrients: Antioxidants, Vitamin C

Raspberry (1 cup):
Potassium: 186mg
Calories: 64
Other Nutrients: Fiber, Antioxidants, Vitamin C

Blackberries (1 cup):
Potassium: 233mg
Calories: 62
Other Nutrients: Fiber, Antioxidants, Vitamin C

Grapefruit (1/2 medium):
Potassium: 166mg
Calories: 52
Other Nutrients: Vitamin A, Vitamin C

Low-Potassium Vegetables

Cabbage (1 cup, shredded):
Potassium: 150mg
Calories: 22
Other Nutrients: Fiber, Vitamin C

Cauliflower (1 cup):
Potassium: 176mg
Calories: 27
Other Nutrients: Fiber, Vitamin C

Bell Peppers (1 medium):
Potassium: 120-200mg
Calories: 25
Other Nutrients: Vitamin A, Vitamin C

Cucumbers (1/2 cup):
Potassium: 80mg
Calories: 8
Other Nutrients: Hydration, Vitamin K

Eggplant (1/2 cup):
Potassium: 120mg
Calories: 13
Other Nutrients: Fiber, Vitamin C

Zucchini (1/2 cup):
Potassium: 150mg
Calories: 13
Other Nutrients: Fiber, Vitamin C

Lettuce (1 cup):
Potassium: 100mg
Calories: 5
Other Nutrients: Vitamin A, Vitamin K

Radishes (1/2 cup):
Potassium: 135mg
Calories: 9
Other Nutrients: Fiber, Vitamin C

Onions (1/2 cup, chopped):
Potassium: 95mg
Calories: 23
Other Nutrients: Fiber, Vitamin C

Carrots (1 medium):
Potassium: 195mg
Calories: 25
Other Nutrients: Vitamin A, Vitamin K

Broccoli (1/2 cup, cooked):
Potassium: 180mg
Calories: 27
Other Nutrients: Fiber, Vitamin C

Green Beans (1/2 cup):
Potassium: 90mg
Calories: 22
Other Nutrients: Fiber, Vitamin C

Cabbage (1 cup, cooked):
Potassium: 135mg
Calories: 44
Other Nutrients: Fiber, Vitamin C

Asparagus (1/2 cup):
Potassium: 135mg
Calories: 20
Other Nutrients: Fiber, Folate

Cauliflower (1/2 cup, cooked):
Potassium: 150mg
Calories: 15
Other Nutrients: Fiber, Vitamin C

Spinach (1/2 cup, cooked):
Potassium: 290mg
Calories: 21
Other Nutrients: Iron, Vitamin A

Cucumber (1 medium):
Potassium: 220mg
Calories: 45
Other Nutrients: Hydration, Vitamin K

Mushrooms (1/2 cup):
Potassium: 150mg
Calories: 10
Other Nutrients: Vitamin D, B-Vitamins

Potatoes (1 medium, boiled):
Potassium: 770mg
Calories: 120
Other Nutrients: Vitamin C, Fiber

Sweet Potatoes (1 medium, baked):
Potassium: 180mg
Calories: 103
Other Nutrients: Vitamin A, Fiber

Low-Potassium Grains and Starches

White Bread (1 slice):
Potassium: 29mg
Calories: 70
Other Nutrients: Carbohydrates

White Rice (1/2 cup, cooked):
Potassium: 35mg
Calories: 103
Other Nutrients: Carbohydrates

Pasta (1/2 cup, cooked):
Potassium: 30mg
Calories: 99
Other Nutrients: Carbohydrates

Cornflakes (1 cup):
Potassium: 30mg
Calories: 100
Other Nutrients: Carbohydrates, Iron

Oats (1/2 cup, cooked):
Potassium: 90mg
Calories: 83
Other Nutrients: Fiber, Carbohydrates

Quinoa (1/2 cup, cooked):
Potassium: 116mg
Calories: 111
Other Nutrients: Protein, Fiber

Barley (1/2 cup, cooked):
Potassium: 119mg
Calories: 97
Other Nutrients: Fiber, Carbohydrates

Couscous (1/2 cup, cooked):
Potassium: 20mg
Calories: 100
Other Nutrients: Carbohydrates

Bulgur (1/2 cup, cooked):
Potassium: 50mg
Calories: 76
Other Nutrients: Fiber, Carbohydrates

Polenta (1/2 cup, cooked):
Potassium: 116mg
Calories: 70
Other Nutrients: Carbohydrates

Millet (1/2 cup, cooked):
Potassium: 60mg
Calories: 104
Other Nutrients: Carbohydrates

White Potatoes (1 medium, boiled):
Potassium: 926mg
Calories: 130
Other Nutrients: Vitamin C, Fiber

Sweet Potatoes (1 medium, baked):
Potassium: 180mg
Calories: 103
Other Nutrients: Vitamin A, Fiber

White Bread (1 roll):
Potassium: 31mg
Calories: 79
Other Nutrients: Carbohydrates

Rice Cakes (1 cake):
Potassium: 0mg
Calories: 35
Other Nutrients: Carbohydrates

Grits (1/2 cup, cooked):
Potassium: 20mg
Calories: 69
Other Nutrients: Carbohydrates

Bagels (1 small):
Potassium: 50mg
Calories: 160
Other Nutrients: Carbohydrates

Tortillas, Corn (1 medium):
Potassium: 15mg
Calories: 52
Other Nutrients: Carbohydrates

Tortillas, Flour (1 medium):
Potassium: 14mg
Calories: 96
Other Nutrients: Carbohydrates

Pretzels, Unsalted (10 pretzels):
Potassium: 15mg
Calories: 127
Other Nutrients: Carbohydrates

Low-Potassium Protein Sources

Chicken (3 ounces, cooked):
Potassium: 220mg
Calories: 165
Other Nutrients: Protein, Vitamin B6

Turkey (3 ounces, cooked):
Potassium: 250mg
Calories: 135
Other Nutrients: Protein, Vitamin B6

Egg Whites (1 large):
Potassium: 55mg
Calories: 17
Other Nutrients: Protein

Tofu (1/2 cup):
Potassium: 140mg
Calories: 94
Other Nutrients: Protein, Calcium

Fish (Salmon, 3 ounces, cooked):
Potassium: 150-200mg
Calories: 155
Other Nutrients: Protein, Omega-3 Fatty Acids

Fish (Tilapia, 3 ounces, cooked):
Potassium: 100mg
Calories: 111
Other Nutrients: Protein

Shrimp (3 ounces, cooked):
Potassium: 150mg
Calories: 101
Other Nutrients: Protein

Crab (3 ounces, cooked):
Potassium: 180mg
Calories: 98
Other Nutrients: Protein

Lobster (3 ounces, cooked):
Potassium: 150mg
Calories: 76
Other Nutrients: Protein

Lean Beef (3 ounces, cooked):
Potassium: 246mg
Calories: 213
Other Nutrients: Protein, Iron

Pork (3 ounces, cooked):
Potassium: 245mg
Calories: 122
Other Nutrients: Protein, Thiamine

Veal (3 ounces, cooked):
Potassium: 220mg
Calories: 156
Other Nutrients: Protein, Vitamin B12

Cottage Cheese (1/2 cup):
Potassium: 69mg
Calories: 110
Other Nutrients: Protein, Calcium

Greek Yogurt, Plain, Non-fat (1/2 cup):
Potassium: 130mg
Calories: 59
Other Nutrients: Protein, Calcium

Milk, Low-Fat (1 cup):
Potassium: 366mg
Calories: 102
Other Nutrients: Protein, Calcium

Cheese, Cheddar (1 ounce):
Potassium: 30mg
Calories: 110
Other Nutrients: Protein, Calcium

Cheese, Swiss (1 ounce):
Potassium: 53mg
Calories: 111
Other Nutrients: Protein, Calcium

Cheese, Mozzarella (Part-Skim, 1 ounce):
Potassium: 54mg
Calories: 72
Other Nutrients: Protein, Calcium

Cheese, Feta (1 ounce):
Potassium: 62mg
Calories: 74
Other Nutrients: Protein, Calcium

Yogurt, Plain, Non-fat (1/2 cup):
Potassium: 150mg
Calories: 50
Other Nutrients: Protein, Calcium

Almond Milk, Unsweetened (1 cup):
Potassium: 150mg
Calories: 30
Other Nutrients: Calcium, Vitamin D

Rice Milk, Unsweetened (1 cup):
Potassium: 10mg
Calories: 70
Other Nutrients: Calcium, Vitamin D

Butter (1 tablespoon):
Potassium: 2mg
Calories: 102
Other Nutrients: Fat

Hard Cheese (Cheddar, 1 ounce):
Potassium: 30mg
Calories: 110
Other Nutrients: Protein, Calcium

Cream Cheese (1 ounce):
Potassium: 28mg
Calories: 50
Other Nutrients: Fat, Protein

Sour Cream, Low-Fat (2 tablespoons):
Potassium: 40mg
Calories: 40
Other Nutrients: Fat, Calcium

Cottage Cheese, Low-Fat (1/2 cup):
Potassium: 69mg
Calories: 110
Other Nutrients: Protein, Calcium

Yogurt, Greek, Plain, Non-fat (1/2 cup):
Potassium: 130mg
Calories: 59
Other Nutrients: Protein, Calcium

Milk, Low-Fat (1 cup):
Potassium: 366mg
Calories: 102
Other Nutrients: Protein, Calcium, Vitamin D

Cream (1 tablespoon):
Potassium: 6mg
Calories: 52
Other Nutrients: Fat

Evaporated Milk, Low-Fat (1 cup):
Potassium: 517mg
Calories: 332
Other Nutrients: Protein, Calcium

Yogurt, Plain, Non-fat (1/2 cup):
Potassium: 150mg
Calories: 50
Other Nutrients: Protein, Calcium

Mozzarella Cheese (Part-Skim, 1 ounce):
Potassium: 54mg
Calories: 72
Other Nutrients: Protein, Calcium

Feta Cheese (1 ounce):
Potassium: 62mg
Calories: 74
Other Nutrients: Protein, Calcium

Soy Milk, Unsweetened (1 cup):
Potassium: 95mg
Calories: 80
Other Nutrients: Protein, Calcium

Coconut Milk, Unsweetened (1 cup):
Potassium: 497mg
Calories: 45
Other Nutrients: Fat

Swiss Cheese (1 ounce):
Potassium: 53mg
Calories: 111
Other Nutrients: Protein, Calcium

Blue Cheese (1 ounce):
Potassium: 32mg
Calories: 100
Other Nutrients: Protein, Calcium

Provolone Cheese (1 ounce):
Potassium: 55mg
Calories: 100
Other Nutrients: Protein, Calcium

Margarine (1 tablespoon):
Potassium: 2mg
Calories: 102
Other Nutrients: Fat

Low-Potassium Snacks

Unsalted Popcorn (1 cup):
Potassium: 20mg
Calories: 31
Other Nutrients: Fiber

Unsalted Pretzels (10 pretzels):
Potassium: 20mg
Calories: 114
Other Nutrients: Carbohydrates

Rice Cakes (1 cake):
Potassium: 20mg
Calories: 35
Other Nutrients: Carbohydrates

Saltine Crackers (5 crackers):
Potassium: 5mg
Calories: 60
Other Nutrients: Carbohydrates

Graham Crackers (2 squares):
Potassium: 20mg
Calories: 60
Other Nutrients: Carbohydrates

Vanilla Wafers (5 cookies):
Potassium: 6mg
Calories: 71
Other Nutrients: Carbohydrates

Animal Crackers (8 crackers):
Potassium: 5mg
Calories: 57
Other Nutrients: Carbohydrates

Pita Bread (1 small, whole):
Potassium: 42mg
Calories: 80
Other Nutrients: Carbohydrates

Melba Toast (4 pieces):
Potassium: 5mg
Calories: 50
Other Nutrients: Carbohydrates

Crispy Rice Cereal (1 cup):
Potassium: 20mg
Calories: 120
Other Nutrients: Carbohydrates

Pretzel Rods (5 rods):
Potassium: 20mg
Calories: 120
Other Nutrients: Carbohydrates

Granola Bar (1 bar):
Potassium: 35mg
Calories: 100
Other Nutrients: Fiber, Carbohydrates

Fruit Leather (1 piece):
Potassium: 30mg
Calories: 50
Other Nutrients: Carbohydrates

Cereal Bar (1 bar):
Potassium: 35mg
Calories: 90
Other Nutrients: Fiber, Carbohydrates

Dried Apple Slices (1/2 cup):
Potassium: 110mg
Calories: 104
Other Nutrients: Fiber

Rice Krispies Treat (1 square):
Potassium: 20mg
Calories: 90
Other Nutrients: Carbohydrates

Pumpkin Seeds (1 ounce):
Potassium: 187mg
Calories: 151
Other Nutrients: Protein

Sunflower Seeds (1 ounce):
Potassium: 90mg
Calories: 204
Other Nutrients: Protein

Apple Sauce, Unsweetened (1/2 cup):
Potassium: 80mg
Calories: 50
Other Nutrients: Fiber

Fruit Cup, Mixed (1 cup, in water):
Potassium: 140mg
Calories: 50
Other Nutrients: Fiber

Low-Potassium Beverages

Water (8 ounces):
Potassium: 0mg
Calories: 0
Other Nutrients: Hydration

Herbal Tea (8 ounces):
Potassium: 0mg
Calories: 0
Other Nutrients: Antioxidants

Black Coffee (8 ounces):
Potassium: 116mg
Calories: 2
Other Nutrients: Caffeine

Green Tea (8 ounces):
Potassium: 0mg
Calories: 0
Other Nutrients: Antioxidants, Caffeine

Clear Soda (8 ounces):
Potassium: 0mg
Calories: Varies (usually low)
Other Nutrients: Carbonation

Apple Juice, Unsweetened (1 cup):
Potassium: 187mg
Calories: 114
Other Nutrients: Vitamin C

Cranberry Juice, Unsweetened (1 cup):
Potassium: 116mg
Calories: 46
Other Nutrients: Antioxidants, Vitamin C

Lemonade, Unsweetened (8 ounces):
Potassium: 0mg
Calories: 5
Other Nutrients: Vitamin C

Grape Juice, Unsweetened (1 cup):
Potassium: 288mg
Calories: 152
Other Nutrients: Antioxidants, Vitamin C

Iced Tea, Unsweetened (8 ounces):
Potassium: 0mg
Calories: 0
Other Nutrients: Antioxidants, Caffeine

Coconut Water (1 cup):
Potassium: 600mg
Calories: 46
Other Nutrients: Hydration, Electrolytes

Almond Milk, Unsweetened (1 cup):
Potassium: 150mg
Calories: 30
Other Nutrients: Calcium, Vitamin D

Rice Milk, Unsweetened (1 cup):
Potassium: 10mg
Calories: 70
Other Nutrients: Calcium, Vitamin D

Sparkling Water (8 ounces):
Potassium: 0mg
Calories: 0
Other Nutrients: Carbonation

Vegetable Juice, Low-Sodium (1 cup):
Potassium: 240mg
Calories: 42
Other Nutrients: Fiber, Vitamins

Tomato Juice, Low-Sodium (1 cup):
Potassium: 556mg
Calories: 41
Other Nutrients: Vitamin C, Lycopene

Ginger Tea (8 ounces):
Potassium: 0mg
Calories: 0
Other Nutrients: Digestive benefits

Orange Juice, Unsweetened (1 cup):
Potassium: 496mg
Calories: 112
Other Nutrients: Vitamin C

Limeade, Unsweetened (8 ounces):
Potassium: 0mg
Calories: 6
Other Nutrients: Vitamin C

Peach Tea, Unsweetened (8 ounces):
Potassium: 0mg
Calories: 0
Other Nutrients: Antioxidants

Low-Potassium Miscellaneous

Butter (1 tablespoon):
Potassium: 2mg
Calories: 102
Other Nutrients: Fat

Margarine (1 tablespoon):
Potassium: 2mg
Calories: 102
Other Nutrients: Fat

Mayonnaise (1 tablespoon):
Potassium: 1mg
Calories: 94
Other Nutrients: Fat

Olive Oil (1 tablespoon):
Potassium: 1mg
Calories: 119
Other Nutrients: Fat

Honey (1 tablespoon):
Potassium: 1mg
Calories: 64
Other Nutrients: Carbohydrates

Maple Syrup (1 tablespoon):
Potassium: 12mg
Calories: 52
Other Nutrients: Carbohydrates

Ketchup (1 tablespoon):
Potassium: 56mg
Calories: 19
Other Nutrients: Carbohydrates

Mustard (1 tablespoon):
Potassium: 5mg
Calories: 3
Other Nutrients: Carbohydrates

Soy Sauce, Low-Sodium (1 tablespoon):
Potassium: 1mg
Calories: 10
Other Nutrients: Sodium (low)

Hot Sauce (1 tablespoon):
Potassium: 2mg
Calories: 1
Other Nutrients: Capsaicin

Vinegar (1 tablespoon):
Potassium: 2mg
Calories: 2
Other Nutrients: Acetic Acid

Pesto Sauce (1 tablespoon):
Potassium: 12mg
Calories: 80
Other Nutrients: Fat, Basil

Tomato Sauce, No Salt Added (1/2 cup):
Potassium: 220mg
Calories: 40
Other Nutrients: Lycopene

Salsa (2 tablespoons):
Potassium: 120mg
Calories: 10
Other Nutrients: Fiber

Horseradish Sauce (1 tablespoon):
Potassium: 10mg
Calories: 7
Other Nutrients: Fiber

Low-Sodium Broth (1 cup):
Potassium: 95mg
Calories: 10
Other Nutrients: Sodium (low)

Low-Sodium Pickles (1 pickle):
Potassium: 15mg
Calories: 5
Other Nutrients: Sodium (low)

Low-Sodium Olives (5 olives):
Potassium: 22mg
Calories: 25
Other Nutrients: Fat, Sodium (low)

Peanut Butter, Unsalted (2 tablespoons):
Potassium: 190mg
Calories: 180
Other Nutrients: Protein

Poppy Seeds (1 tablespoon):
Potassium: 32mg
Calories: 47
Other Nutrients: Fiber, Calcium

Fruits

Apples (1 medium):
Phosphorus: 10mg
Calories: 95
Other Nutrients: Dietary Fiber, Vitamin C

Berries (1 cup, mixed - strawberries, blueberries, raspberries):
Phosphorus: 25mg
Calories: 80
Other Nutrients: Dietary Fiber, Antioxidants

Pineapple (1 cup, diced):
Phosphorus: 13mg
Calories: 82
Other Nutrients: Vitamin C, Manganese

Watermelon (1 cup, diced):
Phosphorus: 11mg
Calories: 46
Other Nutrients: Vitamin A, Vitamin C

Peaches (1 medium):
Phosphorus: 9mg
Calories: 58
Other Nutrients: Vitamin C, Vitamin A

Plums (2 medium):
Phosphorus: 12mg
Calories: 70
Other Nutrients: Dietary Fiber, Vitamin C

Cherries (1 cup):
Phosphorus: 18mg
Calories: 87
Other Nutrients: Dietary Fiber, Vitamin C

Grapes (1 cup, red or green):
Phosphorus: 30mg
Calories: 104
Other Nutrients: Dietary Fiber, Vitamin C

Cantaloupe (1 cup, diced):
Phosphorus: 16mg
Calories: 54
Other Nutrients: Vitamin A, Vitamin C

Oranges (1 medium):
Phosphorus: 15mg
Calories: 62
Other Nutrients: Vitamin C, Dietary Fiber

Vegetables

Cabbage (1 cup, shredded):
Phosphorus: 18mg
Calories: 22
Other Nutrients: Vitamin C, Dietary Fiber

Cauliflower (1 cup, chopped):
Phosphorus: 20mg
Calories: 27
Other Nutrients: Vitamin C, Dietary Fiber

Bell Peppers (1 medium, green):
Phosphorus: 11mg
Calories: 24
Other Nutrients: Vitamin C, Vitamin A

Cucumber (1 medium):
Phosphorus: 21mg
Calories: 45
Other Nutrients: Vitamin K, Vitamin C

Eggplant (1 cup, cubed):
Phosphorus: 9mg
Calories: 20
Other Nutrients: Dietary Fiber, Vitamin C

Zucchini (1 cup, sliced):
Phosphorus: 22mg
Calories: 20
Other Nutrients: Vitamin C, Dietary Fiber

Spinach (1 cup, raw):
Phosphorus: 15mg
Calories: 7
Other Nutrients: Vitamin K, Vitamin A

Kale (1 cup, chopped):
Phosphorus: 28mg
Calories: 33
Other Nutrients: Vitamin K, Vitamin A

Broccoli (1 cup, chopped):
Phosphorus: 38mg
Calories: 55
Other Nutrients: Vitamin C, Dietary Fiber

Green Beans (1 cup, cooked):
Phosphorus: 38mg
Calories: 44
Other Nutrients: Dietary Fiber, Vitamin C

Grains and Starch

White Rice (1 cup, cooked):
Phosphorus: 68mg
Calories: 205
Other Nutrients: Carbohydrates

White Bread (1 slice):
Phosphorus: 23mg
Calories: 79
Other Nutrients: Carbohydrates

Cornflakes (1 cup):
Phosphorus: 48mg
Calories: 100
Other Nutrients: Carbohydrates

Grits (1 cup, cooked):
Phosphorus: 29mg
Calories: 182
Other Nutrients: Carbohydrates

Plain Bagel (1 medium):
Phosphorus: 65mg
Calories: 245
Other Nutrients: Carbohydrates

Rice Cakes (1 cake):
Phosphorus: 6mg
Calories: 35
Other Nutrients: Carbohydrates

Plain Pasta (1 cup, cooked):
Phosphorus: 44mg
Calories: 200
Other Nutrients: Carbohydrates

Oatmeal (1/2 cup, cooked):
Phosphorus: 82mg
Calories: 154
Other Nutrients: Dietary Fiber, Carbohydrates

Plain Popcorn (1 cup, air-popped):
Phosphorus: 37mg
Calories: 31
Other Nutrients: Dietary Fiber, Carbohydrates

Crispy Rice Cereal (1 cup):
Phosphorus: 74mg
Calories: 108
Other Nutrients: Carbohydrates

Chicken (skinless, 3 ounces, roasted):
Phosphorus: 150mg
Calories: 165
Other Nutrients: Protein

Turkey (skinless, 3 ounces, roasted):
Phosphorus: 167mg
Calories: 135
Other Nutrients: Protein

Fish (cod, 3 ounces, baked or grilled):
Phosphorus: 230mg
Calories: 105
Other Nutrients: Protein, Omega-3 Fatty Acids

Eggs (2 large, boiled):
Phosphorus: 124mg
Calories: 155
Other Nutrients: Protein

Tofu (1/2 cup, firm):
Phosphorus: 94mg
Calories: 94
Other Nutrients: Protein

Pork (tenderloin, 3 ounces, roasted):
Phosphorus: 173mg
Calories: 122
Other Nutrients: Protein

Vegetarian Burger Patty (1 patty, commercial):
Phosphorus: 122mg
Calories: 124
Other Nutrients: Protein

Chicken Drumstick (1 drumstick, roasted):
Phosphorus: 138mg
Calories: 76
Other Nutrients: Protein

Cottage Cheese, Low-Fat (1/2 cup):
Phosphorus: 91mg
Calories: 82
Other Nutrients: Protein, Calcium

Salmon (canned, 3 ounces):
Phosphorus: 224mg
Calories: 179
Other Nutrients: Protein, Omega-3 Fatty Acids

Almond Milk, Unsweetened (1 cup):
Phosphorus: 26mg
Calories: 8
Other Nutrients: Calcium, Vitamin D

Rice Milk, Unsweetened (1 cup):
Phosphorus: 39mg
Calories: 70
Other Nutrients: Calcium, Vitamin D

Coconut Milk, Unsweetened (1 cup):
Phosphorus: 50mg
Calories: 45
Other Nutrients: Calcium, Vitamin D

Cottage Cheese, Low-Fat (1/2 cup):
Phosphorus: 91mg
Calories: 82
Other Nutrients: Protein, Calcium

Cream Cheese, Low-Fat (1 tablespoon):
Phosphorus: 14mg
Calories: 35
Other Nutrients: Protein, Calcium

Sour Cream, Low-Fat (2 tablespoons):
Phosphorus: 24mg
Calories: 40
Other Nutrients: Protein, Calcium

Milk, Skim (1 cup):
Phosphorus: 229mg
Calories: 83
Other Nutrients: Protein, Calcium, Vitamin D

Greek Yogurt, Low-Fat (1/2 cup):
Phosphorus: 86mg
Calories: 59
Other Nutrients: Protein, Calcium

Cheese, Mozzarella (1 ounce):
Phosphorus: 183mg
Calories: 72
Other Nutrients: Protein, Calcium

Butter (1 tablespoon):
Phosphorus: 2mg
Calories: 102
Other Nutrients: Fat

Rice Cakes (1 cake):
Phosphorus: 6mg
Calories: 35
Other Nutrients: Carbohydrates

Unsalted Pretzels (10 pretzels):
Phosphorus: 40mg
Calories: 100
Other Nutrients: Carbohydrates

Graham Crackers (2 squares):
Phosphorus: 30mg
Calories: 59
Other Nutrients: Carbohydrates

Animal Crackers (1 ounce):
Phosphorus: 26mg
Calories: 120
Other Nutrients: Carbohydrates

Popcorn (air-popped, 3 cups):
Phosphorus: 50mg
Calories: 93
Other Nutrients: Dietary Fiber

Unsalted Nuts (almonds, 1 ounce):
Phosphorus: 76mg
Calories: 160
Other Nutrients: Protein, Healthy Fats

Fresh Fruit Salad (1 cup):
Phosphorus: Varies by fruit selection
Calories: Varies by fruit selection
Other Nutrients: Vitamins, Dietary Fiber

Low-Phosphorus Crackers (10 crackers):
Phosphorus: 35mg
Calories: 90
Other Nutrients: Carbohydrates

Low-Phosphorus Granola Bar (1 bar):
Phosphorus: 40mg
Calories: 120
Other Nutrients: Carbohydrates, Fiber

Unsalted Sunflower Seeds (1 ounce):
Phosphorus: 150mg
Calories: 160
Other Nutrients: Protein, Healthy Fats

Water (8 ounces):
Phosphorus: 0mg
Calories: 0
Other Nutrients: Hydration

Herbal Tea (8 ounces):
Phosphorus: 0mg
Calories: 0
Other Nutrients: Antioxidants

Black Coffee (8 ounces):
Phosphorus: 2mg
Calories: 2
Other Nutrients: Caffeine

Green Tea (8 ounces):
Phosphorus: 0mg
Calories: 0
Other Nutrients: Antioxidants, Caffeine

Clear Soda (8 ounces):
Phosphorus: 0mg
Calories: Varies (usually low)
Other Nutrients: Carbonation

Unsweetened Almond Milk (1 cup):
Phosphorus: 26mg
Calories: 8
Other Nutrients: Calcium, Vitamin D

Vegetable Juice, Low-Sodium (1 cup):
Phosphorus: 240mg
Calories: 42
Other Nutrients: Fiber, Vitamins

Sparkling Water (8 ounces):
Phosphorus: 0mg
Calories: 0
Other Nutrients: Carbonation

Ginger Tea (8 ounces):
Phosphorus: 0mg
Calories: 0
Other Nutrients: Digestive benefits

Lemonade, Unsweetened (8 ounces):
Phosphorus: 0mg
Calories: 5
Other Nutrients: Vitamin C

Miscellaneous

Butter (1 tablespoon):
Phosphorus: 2mg
Calories: 102
Other Nutrients: Fat

Margarine (1 tablespoon):
Phosphorus: 3mg
Calories: 102
Other Nutrients: Fat

Olive Oil (1 tablespoon):
Phosphorus: 0mg
Calories: 119
Other Nutrients: Fat

Honey (1 tablespoon):
Phosphorus: 1mg
Calories: 64
Other Nutrients: Carbohydrates

Maple Syrup (1 tablespoon):
Phosphorus: 4mg
Calories: 52
Other Nutrients: Carbohydrates

Ketchup (1 tablespoon):
Phosphorus: 5mg
Calories: 19
Other Nutrients: Carbohydrates

Mustard (1 tablespoon):
Phosphorus: 3mg
Calories: 3
Other Nutrients: Carbohydrates

Vinegar (1 tablespoon):
Phosphorus: 0mg
Calories: 2
Other Nutrients: Acetic Acid

Pesto Sauce (1 tablespoon):
Phosphorus: 4mg
Calories: 80
Other Nutrients: Fat, Basil

Salsa (2 tablespoons):
Phosphorus: 20mg
Calories: 10
Other Nutrients: Fiber

Kidney-Friendly Breakfast Options

Oatmeal with Fresh Berries:
Oatmeal (1/2 cup, cooked)
Phosphorus: 45mg
Sodium: 0mg
Potassium: 110mg
Calories: 150

Fresh Berries (1/2 cup)
Phosphorus: 15mg
Sodium: 1mg
Potassium: 90mg
Calories: Varies

Egg White Omelette with Vegetables:
Egg Whites (2 eggs)
Phosphorus: 124mg
Sodium: 148mg
Potassium: 206mg
Calories: 34

Mixed Vegetables (bell peppers, onions, spinach)
Phosphorus: Varies
Sodium: Varies

Potassium: Varies
Calories: Varies
Greek Yogurt Parfait:

Greek Yogurt, Low-Fat (1/2 cup)
Phosphorus: 86mg
Sodium: 50mg
Potassium: 110mg
Calories: 59

Fresh Fruit (berries, banana slices)
Phosphorus: Varies
Sodium: Varies
Potassium: Varies
Calories: Varies

Whole Grain Toast with Avocado:
Whole Grain Toast (1 slice)
Phosphorus: 37mg
Sodium: 88mg
Potassium: 63mg
Calories: 69

Avocado (1/4 medium)
Phosphorus: 22mg
Sodium: 1mg
Potassium: 195mg
Calories: 60

Smoothie with Spinach and Berries:
Spinach (1 cup, fresh)
Phosphorus: 15mg
Sodium: 24mg
Potassium: 167mg
Calories: 7

Mixed Berries (1/2 cup)
Phosphorus: 15mg
Sodium: 1mg
Potassium: 90mg
Calories: Varies

Low-Potassium Pancakes with Maple Syrup:
Low-Potassium Pancake Mix (1 serving)
Phosphorus: Varies
Sodium: Varies
Potassium: Varies
Calories: Varies

Maple Syrup (2 tablespoons)
Phosphorus: 8mg
Sodium: 2mg
Potassium: 42mg
Calories: 100

Cottage Cheese with Pineapple:
Cottage Cheese, Low-Fat (1/2 cup)
Phosphorus: 91mg
Sodium: 325mg
Potassium: 117mg

Calories: 82

Pineapple Chunks (1/2 cup)
Phosphorus: 11mg
Sodium: 0mg
Potassium: 90mg
Calories: 41

Low-Sodium Breakfast Burrito:
Scrambled Eggs (2 eggs)
Phosphorus: 124mg
Sodium: 148mg
Potassium: 206mg
Calories: 136

Low-Sodium Salsa (2 tablespoons)
Phosphorus: 20mg
Sodium: 10mg
Potassium: 80mg
Calories: 10

Whole Wheat Tortilla (1 medium)
Phosphorus: 67mg
Sodium: 147mg
Potassium: 108mg
Calories: 138

Quinoa Breakfast Bowl:
Quinoa, Cooked (1/2 cup)
Phosphorus: 66mg
Sodium: 5mg

Potassium: 115mg
Calories: 111

Almond Milk, Unsweetened (1/2 cup)
Phosphorus: 13mg
Sodium: 135mg
Potassium: 180mg
Calories: 13

Sliced Banana (1/2 medium)
Phosphorus: 13mg
Sodium: 1mg
Potassium: 211mg
Calories: 53

Low-Phosphorus Bran Muffin with Cream Cheese:
Low-Phosphorus Bran Muffin (1 medium)
Phosphorus: Varies
Sodium: Varies
Potassium: Varies
Calories: Varies

Cream Cheese, Low-Fat (1 tablespoon)
Phosphorus: 14mg
Sodium: 38mg
Potassium: 27mg
Calories: 29

Grilled Chicken Salad:
Grilled Chicken Breast (3 ounces)
Phosphorus: 220mg
Sodium: 74mg
Potassium: 220mg
Calories: 142

Mixed Greens (2 cups)
Phosphorus: 30mg
Sodium: 10mg
Potassium: 260mg
Calories: Varies

Cherry Tomatoes (1/2 cup)
Phosphorus: 11mg
Sodium: 6mg
Potassium: 146mg
Calories: 15

Balsamic Vinaigrette Dressing (2 tablespoons)
Phosphorus: 10mg
Sodium: 80mg
Potassium: 30mg
Calories: 70

Vegetable Stir-Fry with Tofu:
Tofu (1/2 cup)
Phosphorus: 94mg
Sodium: 3mg
Potassium: 140mg
Calories: 94

Mixed Vegetables (bell peppers, broccoli, carrots) (1 cup)
Phosphorus: Varies
Sodium: Varies
Potassium: Varies
Calories: Varies

Brown Rice (1/2 cup, cooked)
Phosphorus: 66mg
Sodium: 2mg
Potassium: 86mg
Calories: 108

Salmon Wrap with Avocado:
Grilled Salmon (3 ounces)
Phosphorus: 230mg
Sodium: 50mg
Potassium: 430mg
Calories: 180

Whole Wheat Wrap (1 medium)
Phosphorus: 124mg
Sodium: 330mg
Potassium: 100mg

Calories: 170

Avocado Slices (1/4 medium)
Phosphorus: 22mg
Sodium: 1mg
Potassium: 195mg
Calories: 60

Turkey and Veggie Sandwich:
Turkey Breast, Low-Sodium (3 ounces)
Phosphorus: 150mg
Sodium: 60mg
Potassium: 240mg
Calories: 90

Whole Grain Bread (2 slices)
Phosphorus: 74mg
Sodium: 150mg
Potassium: 150mg
Calories: 160

Lettuce, Tomato, Onion (1/2 cup)
Phosphorus: Varies
Sodium: Varies
Potassium: Varies
Calories: Varies

Quinoa and Black Bean Bowl:
Quinoa, Cooked (1/2 cup)
Phosphorus: 66mg
Sodium: 5mg
Potassium: 115mg
Calories: 111

Black Beans, Low-Sodium (1/2 cup)
Phosphorus: 45mg
Sodium: 5mg
Potassium: 220mg
Calories: 109

Salsa (2 tablespoons)
Phosphorus: 20mg
Sodium: 10mg
Potassium: 80mg
Calories: 10

Egg Salad Lettuce Wraps:
Hard-Boiled Eggs (2 large)
Phosphorus: 248mg
Sodium: 140mg
Potassium: 126mg
Calories: 156

Lettuce Leaves (4 large)
Phosphorus: Varies
Sodium: Varies
Potassium: Varies
Calories: Varies

Dijon Mustard (1 teaspoon)
Phosphorus: 5mg
Sodium: 45mg
Potassium: 15mg
Calories: 5

Vegetarian Lentil Soup:
Lentils, Cooked (1/2 cup)
Phosphorus: 93mg
Sodium: 1mg
Potassium: 239mg
Calories: 115

Carrots, Celery, Onion (1/2 cup)
Phosphorus: Varies
Sodium: Varies
Potassium: Varies
Calories: Varies

Low-Sodium Vegetable Broth (1 cup)
Phosphorus: 30mg
Sodium: 140mg
Potassium: 210mg
Calories: 20

Chickpea Salad with Feta:
Chickpeas, Canned, Drained (1/2 cup)
Phosphorus: 70mg
Sodium: 144mg
Potassium: 143mg
Calories: 134

Cucumber, Tomato, Red Onion (1/2 cup)
Phosphorus: Varies
Sodium: Varies
Potassium: Varies
Calories: Varies

Feta Cheese, Crumbled (2 tablespoons)
Phosphorus: 40mg
Sodium: 140mg
Potassium: 20mg
Calories: 50

Baked Chicken with Sweet Potatoes:
Baked Chicken Thigh (3 ounces)
Phosphorus: 180mg
Sodium: 75mg
Potassium: 228mg
Calories: 166

Sweet Potato, Baked (1 medium)
Phosphorus: 70mg
Sodium: 15mg
Potassium: 542mg
Calories: 103

Steamed Broccoli (1/2 cup)
Phosphorus: 20mg
Sodium: 30mg
Potassium: 180mg
Calories: 27

Low-Sodium Vegetable and Chicken Wrap:
Grilled Chicken Breast (3 ounces)
Phosphorus: 220mg
Sodium: 74mg
Potassium: 220mg
Calories: 142

Whole Wheat Wrap (1 medium)
Phosphorus: 124mg
Sodium: 330mg
Potassium: 100mg
Calories: 170

Mixed Vegetables (bell peppers, cucumber, lettuce) (1/2 cup)
Phosphorus: Varies
Sodium: Varies
Potassium: Varies
Calories: Varies

Baked Salmon with Lemon and Herbs:
Baked Salmon Fillet (3 ounces)
Phosphorus: 230mg
Sodium: 50mg
Potassium: 430mg
Calories: 180

Lemon and Herbs (for seasoning)
Phosphorus: Varies
Sodium: Varies
Potassium: Varies
Calories: Varies

Steamed Asparagus (1/2 cup)
Phosphorus: 15mg
Sodium: 0mg
Potassium: 135mg
Calories: 20

Vegetarian Quinoa Bowl:
Quinoa, Cooked (1/2 cup)
Phosphorus: 66mg
Sodium: 5mg
Potassium: 115mg
Calories: 111

Black Beans, Low-Sodium (1/2 cup)
Phosphorus: 45mg
Sodium: 5mg
Potassium: 220mg
Calories: 109

Roasted Vegetables (bell peppers, zucchini, cherry tomatoes) (1/2 cup)
Phosphorus: Varies
Sodium: Varies
Potassium: Varies
Calories: Varies

Grilled Chicken Breast with Roasted Sweet Potatoes:
Grilled Chicken Breast (3 ounces)
Phosphorus: 220mg
Sodium: 74mg
Potassium: 220mg
Calories: 142

Sweet Potato, Roasted (1 medium)
Phosphorus: 70mg
Sodium: 15mg
Potassium: 542mg
Calories: 103

Steamed Green Beans (1/2 cup)
Phosphorus: 20mg
Sodium: 2mg
Potassium: 88mg

Calories: 17

Vegetable and Tofu Stir-Fry:
Tofu, Extra Firm (1/2 cup)
Phosphorus: 94mg
Sodium: 3mg
Potassium: 140mg
Calories: 94

Mixed Vegetables (broccoli, carrots, snow peas) (1 cup)
Phosphorus: Varies
Sodium: Varies
Potassium: Varies
Calories: Varies

Brown Rice, Cooked (1/2 cup)
Phosphorus: 66mg
Sodium: 2mg
Potassium: 86mg
Calories: 108

Lentil Soup with Spinach:
Lentils, Cooked (1/2 cup)
Phosphorus: 93mg
Sodium: 1mg
Potassium: 239mg
Calories: 115

Spinach (1 cup, fresh)
Phosphorus: 15mg
Sodium: 24mg
Potassium: 167mg
Calories: 7

Low-Sodium Vegetable Broth (1 cup)
Phosphorus: 30mg
Sodium: 140mg
Potassium: 210mg
Calories: 20

Turkey and Vegetable Skewers:
Turkey Breast, Cubed (3 ounces)
Phosphorus: 150mg
Sodium: 60mg
Potassium: 240mg
Calories: 90

Bell Peppers and Cherry Tomatoes (1/2 cup)
Phosphorus: Varies
Sodium: Varies
Potassium: Varies
Calories: Varies

Quinoa, Cooked (1/2 cup)
Phosphorus: 66mg
Sodium: 5mg
Potassium: 115mg
Calories: 111

Baked Chicken with Lemon and Rosemary:
Baked Chicken Thigh (3 ounces)
Phosphorus: 180mg
Sodium: 75mg
Potassium: 228mg
Calories: 166

Lemon and Rosemary (for seasoning)
Phosphorus: Varies
Sodium: Varies
Potassium: Varies
Calories: Varies

Mashed Cauliflower (1/2 cup)
Phosphorus: 30mg
Sodium: 30mg
Potassium: 288mg
Calories: 66

Salmon and Asparagus Foil Packets:
Salmon Fillet (3 ounces)
Phosphorus: 230mg
Sodium: 50mg
Potassium: 430mg
Calories: 180

Asparagus Spears (1/2 cup)
Phosphorus: 15mg
Sodium: 0mg
Potassium: 135mg
Calories: 20

Olive Oil, Lemon, and Garlic (for seasoning)
Phosphorus: Varies
Sodium: Varies
Potassium: Varies
Calories: Varies

Vegetarian Stuffed Bell Peppers:
Quinoa, Cooked (1/2 cup)
Phosphorus: 66mg
Sodium: 5mg
Potassium: 115mg
Calories: 111

Black Beans, Low-Sodium (1/2 cup)
Phosphorus: 45mg
Sodium: 5mg
Potassium: 220mg
Calories: 109

Bell Peppers, Stuffed and Baked (1 medium)
Phosphorus: Varies
Sodium: Varies
Potassium: Varies
Calories: Varies

Pasta with Tomato and Basil Sauce:
Whole Wheat Pasta (1/2 cup, cooked)
Phosphorus: 45mg
Sodium: 0mg
Potassium: 80mg
Calories: 87

Tomato and Basil Sauce (1/2 cup)
Phosphorus: 25mg
Sodium: 330mg
Potassium: 300mg
Calories: 70

Grated Parmesan Cheese (1 tablespoon)
Phosphorus: 21mg
Sodium: 76mg
Potassium: 10mg
Calories: 22

Kidney-Friendly Snacks and Desserts

Apple Slices with Almond Butter:
Apple Slices (1 medium)
Phosphorus: 10mg
Sodium: 0mg
Potassium: 195mg
Calories: 95

Almond Butter (1 tablespoon)
Phosphorus: 50mg
Sodium: 0mg
Potassium: 80mg
Calories: 98

Greek Yogurt with Berries:
Greek Yogurt, Low-Fat (1/2 cup)
Phosphorus: 86mg
Sodium: 50mg
Potassium: 110mg
Calories: 59

Mixed Berries (1/2 cup)
Phosphorus: 15mg
Sodium: 1mg
Potassium: 90mg
Calories: Varies

Banana and Walnut Muffins (Low-Phosphorus):
Banana (1 medium)
Phosphorus: 27mg
Sodium: 1mg
Potassium: 422mg
Calories: 105

Chopped Walnuts (2 tablespoons)
Phosphorus: 34mg
Sodium: 0mg
Potassium: 74mg
Calories: 93

Rice Cake with Avocado:
Rice Cake (1 plain)
Phosphorus: 15mg
Sodium: 0mg

Potassium: 0mg
Calories: 35

Avocado (1/4 medium)
Phosphorus: 22mg
Sodium: 1mg
Potassium: 195mg
Calories: 60

Low-Sodium Popcorn:
Air-Popped Popcorn (3 cups)
Phosphorus: 84mg
Sodium: 0mg
Potassium: 93mg
Calories: 93

Olive Oil Spray and Herbs (for seasoning)
Phosphorus: Varies
Sodium: Varies
Potassium: Varies
Calories: Varies

Peach and Cottage Cheese Bowl:
Cottage Cheese, Low-Fat (1/2 cup)
Phosphorus: 91mg
Sodium: 325mg
Potassium: 117mg
Calories: 82

Fresh Peach Slices (1 medium)
Phosphorus: 11mg
Sodium: 0mg
Potassium: 285mg
Calories: 59

Frozen Banana Bites:
Banana Slices (1 medium)
Phosphorus: 27mg
Sodium: 1mg
Potassium: 422mg
Calories: 105

Dark Chocolate (1 ounce, melted)
Phosphorus: 50mg
Sodium: 0mg
Potassium: 116mg
Calories: 155

Low-Phosphorus Jello Cups:
Sugar-Free Jello (1/2 cup)
Phosphorus: 5mg
Sodium: 40mg
Potassium: 7mg
Calories: 10

Whipped Topping (2 tablespoons)
Phosphorus: 10mg
Sodium: 0mg
Potassium: 5mg
Calories: 25

Cherry Tomato and Mozzarella Skewers:
Cherry Tomatoes (1/2 cup)
Phosphorus: 11mg
Sodium: 6mg
Potassium: 146mg
Calories: 15

Mozzarella Balls (2 ounces)
Phosphorus: 110mg
Sodium: 160mg
Potassium: 50mg
Calories: 140

Low-Phosphorus Popsicles:
Fruit Juice Popsicles (1 popsicle)
Phosphorus: 5mg
Sodium: 0mg
Potassium: 20mg
Calories: 20

Fresh Fruit Chunks (for added flavor)
Phosphorus: Varies
Sodium: Varies
Potassium: Varies
Calories: Varies

SHOPPING LIST

1. Chicken breast
2. Turkey
3. Fish (salmon, cod)
4. Eggs
5. Tofu
6. Low-sodium canned beans
7. Cauliflower
8. Broccoli
9. Green beans
10. Bell peppers
11. Apples
12. Berries (blueberries, strawberries)
13. Pineapple
14. Cherries
15. White bread
16. Rice cakes
17. Low-sodium pasta
18. Quinoa
19. Olive oil
20. Canola oil
21. Butter (in moderation)
22. Low-fat mayonnaise
23. Low-sodium soy sauce
24. Vinegar
25. Garlic
26. Onions
27. Low-sodium chicken broth
28. Low-sodium vegetable broth
29. Oatmeal
30. Cream of wheat

31. Low-sodium cereal
32. Low-fat milk
33. Greek yogurt
34. Low-fat cheese
35. Low-sodium cottage cheese
36. Low-sodium hummus
37. Mustard
38. Fresh herbs (parsley, basil)
39. Cabbage
40. Lettuce
41. Watermelon
42. Cucumber
43. Zucchini
44. Straw mushrooms
45. Low-potassium fruit juices
46. Cranberry juice
47. Raspberry jam (without added phosphorus)
48. Honey
49. Agave syrup
50. Unsweetened applesauce
51. Ginger
52. Brown rice
53. Red peppers
54. Cherry tomatoes
55. Low-sodium ketchup
56. Low-sodium salsa
57. Low-sodium marinara sauce
58. Low-sodium canned tomatoes
59. Sweet potatoes
60. Turnips
61. Radishes
62. Low-sodium canned corn

     KIDNEY DISEASE DIET FOODS CHART FOR SENIORS
ON STAGE 3

63. Green onions
64. Eggplant
65. Low-sodium olives
66. Low-sodium pickles
67. Water chestnuts
68. Low-sodium salad dressing
69. Pears
70. Peaches
71. Plums
72. Nectarines
73. Low-sodium nuts (almonds, cashews)
74. Low-sodium nut butter
75. Low-sodium popcorn
76. Low-sodium pretzels
77. Gingersnaps (low-sodium)
78. Vanilla wafers (low-sodium)
79. Angel food cake
80. Popsicles (homemade, low-sodium)
81. Hard candies (peppermints, lemon drops)
82. Sherbet
83. Cilantro
84. Dill
85. Low-sodium Worcestershire sauce
86. Basil pesto
87. Lemons
88. Peppermint tea
89. Lemonade
90. Unsalted rice cakes
91. Low-sodium beef broth
92. Unsweetened almond milk
93. Low-sodium vegetable juice
94. Low-sodium tomato juice

  KIDNEY DISEASE DIET FOODS CHART FOR SENIORS ON STAGE 3

95. Low-sodium cranberry sauce
96. Lemon zest
97. Lime zest
98. Low-sodium hot sauce
99. Low-sodium teriyaki sauce
100.   Herb-infused water

CONCLUSION

In conclusion, the kidney disease diet for seniors in Stage 3 Chronic Kidney Disease (CKD) stands as a pivotal tool in the management and maintenance of health for this specific demographic. The carefully curated food list, which emphasizes moderation and balance, plays a crucial role in supporting kidney function, managing symptoms, and promoting overall well-being among older individuals facing this stage of kidney disease.

Understanding the unique challenges presented by Stage 3 CKD, where the kidneys demonstrate moderate impairment, underscores the importance of adopting a specialized dietary approach. While seniors at this stage may not always exhibit noticeable symptoms, the proactive implementation of a kidney-friendly diet becomes paramount in mitigating further damage to the kidneys, regulating electrolyte balance, and controlling blood pressure.

The key components of the kidney disease diet, including sodium regulation, potassium management, phosphorus control, protein moderation, and fluid balance, offer a comprehensive strategy to address the specific needs of seniors with Stage 3 CKD. By adhering to these dietary guidelines, individuals in this stage can actively contribute to slowing the progression of kidney dysfunction and minimizing the risk of associated complications.

Furthermore, the emphasis on an individualized approach recognizes the uniqueness of each senior's health profile, taking into account personal preferences, cultural considerations, and specific health conditions. Consulting with a registered dietitian remains integral to tailoring the kidney disease diet to the individual, ensuring that it aligns with their needs, enhances their quality of life, and supports their overall health journey.

In the journey of managing Stage 3 CKD, the kidney disease diet emerges as a proactive and empowering tool, empowering seniors to take charge of their health and well-being. Regular communication with healthcare professionals, including dietitians and nephrologists, ensures ongoing adjustments to the dietary plan based on individual health status, providing seniors with the knowledge and support they need to thrive despite the challenges of Stage 3 CKD. Through this holistic and personalized approach, seniors can embrace a kidney-friendly lifestyle that fosters a sense of control, resilience, and improved health in their golden years.

Dear Cherished Readers

I trust this book has served as a wellspring of inspiration, solace, and valuable insights for you. Each recipe was crafted with love, meticulous attention to detail, and a profound understanding of effective utilization of the Kidney Disease Stage 3 food list for seniors, ensuring wholesome and nutritious meals.

Your reviews, experiences, and insights are invaluable. Every evaluation propels me to enhance and tailor my work to better cater to your needs. Let's engage in a meaningful discussion—a dialogue that transcends the written words, forging a deeper connection. Your thoughts are the driving force behind continuous improvement.

Warm regards,

Felicia O. Pace

To explore additional evidence-based and approved nutrition books similar to this one, please feel free to visit my Amazon store HERE

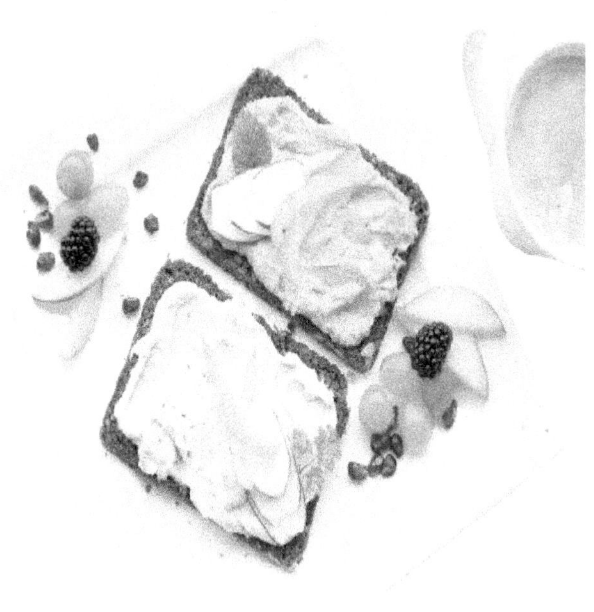

     KIDNEY DISEASE DIET FOODS CHART FOR SENIORS ON STAGE 3

www.ingramcontent.com/pod-product-compliance
Lightning Source LLC
Chambersburg PA
CBHW070758260726
48660CB00005B/1683